BRONCHIECTASIS

A Beginner's 3-Step Guide on Managing Bronchiectasis Through Natural Methods and Diet, With Sample Recipes and a Meal Plan

Patrick Marshwell

mindplusfood

mf

Copyright © 2022 Patrick Marshwell

All rights reserved

No part of this book may be reproduced, or stored in a retrieval system, or transmitted in any form or by any means, electronic, mechanical, photocopying, recording, or otherwise, without express written permission of the publisher.

Printed in the United States of America

CONTENTS

Title Page
Copyright
Disclaimer
Introduction ... 1
What Is Bronchiectasis? ... 3
Symptoms of Bronchiectasis ... 5
Diagnosing and Treating Bronchiectasis ... 7
A 3-Step Guide on Managing Bronchiectasis ... 9
Sample Meals ... 17
Conclusion ... 33
FAQ about Bronchiectasis ... 34
Key Takeaways ... 37
References ... 38

DISCLAIMER

By reading this disclaimer, you are accepting the terms of the disclaimer in full. If you disagree with this disclaimer, please do not read the guide.

All of the content within this guide is provided for informational and educational purposes only, and should not be accepted as independent medical or other professional advice. The author is not a doctor, physician, nurse, mental health provider, or registered nutritionist/dietician. Therefore, using and reading this guide does not establish any form of a physician-patient relationship.

Always consult with a physician or another qualified health provider with any issues or questions you might have regarding any sort of medical condition. Do not ever disregard any qualified professional medical advice or delay seeking that advice because of anything you have read in this guide. The information in this guide is not intended to be any sort of medical advice and should not be used in lieu of any medical advice by a licensed and qualified medical professional.

The information in this guide has been compiled from a variety of known sources. However, the author cannot attest to or guarantee the accuracy of each source and thus should not be held liable for any errors or omissions.

You acknowledge that the publisher of this guide will not be held liable for any loss or damage of any kind incurred as a result of this guide or the reliance on any information provided within this guide. You acknowledge and agree that you assume all risk and responsibility for any action you undertake in response to the information in this guide.

Using this guide does not guarantee any particular result (e.g., weight loss or a cure). By reading this guide, you acknowledge that there are no guarantees to any specific outcome or results you can expect.

All product names, diet plans, or names used in this guide are for identification purposes only and are the property of their respective owners. The use of these names does not imply endorsement. All other trademarks cited herein are the property of their respective owners.

Where applicable, this guide is not intended to be a substitute for the original work of this diet plan and is, at most, a supplement to the original work for this diet plan and never a direct substitute. This guide is a personal expression of the facts of that diet plan.

Where applicable, persons shown in the cover images are stock photography models and the publisher has obtained the rights to use the images through license agreements with third-party stock image companies.

INTRODUCTION

Bronchiectasis is a lung condition that lasts for a long time and is chronic. In the United States alone, it's believed that about 500,000 of the population suffer from it. As for the older demographic, out of 150 people aged 75 and older, one of them has bronchiectasis. It creates inflammation in the airways and can damage them. It may then become difficult to breathe as a result of the accumulation of mucus that this may cause. Bronchiectasis has been linked to an increased likelihood of contracting various respiratory illnesses.

There is currently no known treatment that will reverse the effects of bronchiectasis; however, there are medicines that can assist to manage the condition and alleviate its symptoms. These include going to frequent physiotherapy sessions, taking antibiotics to prevent infections, and adopting adjustments to one's lifestyle such as giving up smoking and minimizing exposure to irritants. Other treatments may also be prescribed.

People who have bronchiectasis should also focus on maintaining a nutritious diet, as this can assist to strengthen the immune system and decrease inflammation. Antioxidant foods, foods high in omega-3 fatty acids, and foods high in vitamin C are particularly good for one's health.

Bronchiectasis is an illness that can be debilitating, but it is possible to live a life that is relatively normal with the proper therapy and by making adjustments to one's lifestyle.

In this beginner's quick start guide, we will discuss bronchiectasis in more detail, including its causes, symptoms, and treatment options. We will also provide a 3-step guide on how to manage the condition through diet and lifestyle changes.

You will discover...
- All there is to know about bronchiectasis
- Symptoms and risk factors of bronchiectasis
- Diagnosing and treating the condition
- Different ways to manage bronchiectasis
- Diet plan that's bronchiectasis friendly

WHAT IS BRONCHIECTASIS?

Bronchiectasis is a long-term, chronic lung condition that causes inflammation and damage to the airways, leading to a build-up of mucus, making breathing difficult. You may also be at an increased risk of developing other respiratory infections. Furthermore, the condition can be debilitating, making it difficult to carry out everyday activities.

After undergoing a series of diagnostic procedures, such as a chest x-ray, CT scan, and sputum culture, a pulmonologist (also known as a lung specialist) will often make the diagnosis of bronchiectasis in a patient.

Causes
It's not actually possible to pinpoint the exact cause of bronchiectasis. According to some studies, the condition results from either an injury to the airway walls or from a lung infection such as cystic fibrosis (CF). However, there are also other cases not linked to CF, also called idiopathic bronchiectasis. According to Cleveland Clinic, some idiopathic bronchiectasis cases may include or have resulted from the following:
- Severe lung infection that caused damage previously
- Conditions that affect the immune system
- Things like fluids, food, or stomach acid that go into the

lungs through aspirating
- Airways obstructed by a tumor or other objects that were inhaled
- Some genetic diseases like alpha-1 antitrypsin deficiency and primary ciliary dyskinesia
- A condition called allergic bronchopulmonary aspergillosis, which is caused by an allergy to a specific kind of fungus
- Crohn's disease, rheumatoid arthritis, Sjogren's syndrome, and other conditions

Risk Factors

Aside from possible causes, some people may also risk suffering from bronchiectasis due to having the following conditions:

- *Cystic fibrosis* - is an inherited condition that causes the body to produce abnormally thick and sticky mucus. This can lead to blockages in the airways and a build-up of bacteria, which can damage the lungs.

- *Chronic obstructive pulmonary disease (COPD)* - is a group of conditions that make it difficult to breathe, including emphysema and chronic bronchitis.

- *Asthma* - a condition that causes the airways to narrow and swell, making it difficult to breathe.

- *Autoimmune diseases* - conditions that occur when the body's immune system attacks healthy tissue, such as rheumatoid arthritis and lupus.

- *Infections* - such as tuberculosis (TB) and pneumonia. Previous lung surgery or radiotherapy to the chest.

Bronchiectasis may be caused by a variety of factors, including genetics, smoking, respiratory infections, environmental pollutants, and autoimmune diseases. People with certain risk factors, such as a family history of bronchiectasis, are more likely to develop the condition.

SYMPTOMS OF BRONCHIECTASIS

Bronchiectasis is a progressive condition, which means that it will get worse over time if it is not treated. In the early stages, the symptoms may be mild and only occur occasionally. However, as the condition progresses, the symptoms will become more severe and can occur more frequently.

A persistent cough that is accompanied by the production of mucus is the most typical sign of bronchiectasis. Among the other symptoms are:

- <u>Shortness of breath</u> - Shortness of breath is one of the most common bronchiectasis symptoms. You may feel out of breath after carrying out everyday activities, such as walking up the stairs. This is because the widening of your airways makes it harder for you to move air in and out of your lungs.

- <u>Wheezing</u> - You may experience wheezing when you have bronchiectasis. This is due to the build-up of mucus in your lungs, which narrows your airways and makes it difficult to breathe.

- <u>Chest pain</u> - You may experience tightness or pain in your chest. This is caused by the inflammation of your airways and the build-up of mucus.

- _Fatigue_ - You may feel tired and low in energy. This is because your body is working harder to breathe. The extra effort your body expends can leave you feeling fatigued.

- _Weight loss_ - As the condition progresses, you may start to lose weight. This is because it becomes increasingly difficult to digest and absorb nutrients from food. In addition, bronchiectasis can lead to a build-up of mucus in the lungs, making it difficult to breathe. This can result in loss of appetite and fatigue, both of which can lead to weight loss.

- _Frequent respiratory infections_ - If you have bronchiectasis, you might experience frequent respiratory infections, such as bronchitis and pneumonia.

- _Clubbing of the fingers and toes_ - You may experience clubbing of the fingers and toes if you have bronchiectasis. This is when the nails become thickened and curved, and usually only occurs in severe cases. If you notice this symptom, it is important to see a doctor so that they can determine the cause and provide treatment.

You may also have a cough that produces mucus. The mucus may be thick and difficult to expel. You may notice that you're coughing up blood, or that you have increased respiratory infections.

Visit your primary care provider as soon as possible if you notice any of these symptoms; they will be able to diagnose your problem and get you started on the treatment that is most appropriate for it.

DIAGNOSING AND TREATING BRONCHIECTASIS

If you have a cough that has lasted for more than three weeks, produces mucus or blood, or both, you should see a doctor. Insufficiency of breath, difficulty breathing, recurring lung infections, and exhaustion are some of the additional symptoms that may be indicative of bronchiectasis.

Your doctor will likely order a chest X-ray and a CT scan to confirm the diagnosis. They may also order a bronchoscopy, during which a small camera is inserted down your throat to get a closer look at your airways. A bronchoscopy can also be used to collect a sample of mucus from your lungs, which can be tested for bacteria.

Once bronchiectasis is confirmed, your doctor will work with you to develop a treatment plan. This may include antibiotics to clear lung infections, inhaled medications to open up the airways, and daily chest physiotherapy to help remove mucus from the lungs. In severe cases, surgery may be necessary to remove damaged sections of the lungs.

- Antibiotics - Antibiotics may be prescribed to prevent lung infections. In some cases, they may also be used to treat an active infection.

- Physiotherapy - Regular physiotherapy is an important part of treatment for bronchiectasis. It helps to clear mucus from the lungs and prevent it from building up. Physiotherapy can also help to improve your breathing and overall fitness.

The majority of people who have bronchiectasis can live relatively normal lives if they receive the appropriate treatment. On the other hand, it is essential that you continue to cooperate with your physician in order to manage the condition and prevent flare-ups.

Because pneumonia and other respiratory infections can be dangerous for people who have bronchiectasis, it is important to ensure that your vaccinations are up to date at all times. Additionally, the best way to prevent further damage to the lungs is to give up smoking and stay away from environments with secondhand smoke.

A 3-STEP GUIDE ON MANAGING BRONCHIECTASIS

If you have been diagnosed with bronchiectasis, it is important to begin managing the condition as soon as possible. While there is no cure for bronchiectasis, there are many natural methods and dietary changes that can help lessen the symptoms and improve your quality of life. In this section, we will discuss the 3-step guide on managing Bronchiectasis through natural methods and diet.

Step One: Identifying and Avoiding Triggers
Bronchiectasis is a chronic lung condition that causes your airways to become widened and damaged. This can lead to difficulty breathing, coughing, and increased mucus production.

The main goal of bronchiectasis management is to prevent or reduce the symptoms of the condition. To do this, it is important to identify and avoid triggers that can exacerbate your condition. Some common triggers include tobacco smoke, air pollution, infection, and allergens. If you have bronchiectasis, it is important to take steps to avoid these triggers and keep your lungs healthy.

- *Respiratory infections* - The best way to manage

bronchiectasis is to identify and avoid triggers that can make your symptoms worse. Common triggers include respiratory infections, such as influenza and pneumonia. Be sure to get vaccinated against these infections to help reduce your risk.

- *Air pollution* - Air pollution is a common trigger for bronchiectasis flare-ups. If you live in an area with high levels of air pollution, try to avoid spending time outdoors, and if possible, stay indoors with the windows closed. You may also want to consider investing in an air purifier to help improve the quality of the air in your home.

- *Smoke* - one of the most common triggers of bronchiectasis is smoke. If you smoke, now is the time to quit. Smoking is the leading cause of bronchiectasis. Avoid secondhand smoke as well.

- *Certain medications* - Some medications, such as beta-blockers and angiotensin-converting enzyme inhibitors, can worsen bronchiectasis. If you are taking any of these medications, talk to your doctor about alternatives.

- *Dry air* - Dry air can irritate the lungs and lead to mucus buildup. If you live in an area with dry air, use a humidifier in your home to add moisture to the air.

Keeping track of what you were doing when you had an exacerbation can help you to identify your triggers. Once you know what your triggers are, you can take steps to avoid them.

Step Two: Improving Lung Function
While there is no cure for bronchiectasis, there are natural methods that can help to improve lung function and reduce symptoms. These include:

Deep breathing exercises
Many people find that deep breathing exercises can help to

improve their lung function and prevent mucus buildup. The reason for this is that deep breathing helps to increase the amount of oxygen in the blood, which in turn helps to loosen mucus and clear the airways.

In addition, deep breathing helps to strengthen the muscles around the lungs, making it easier to breathe. For best results, it is important to practice deep breathing regularly and to make sure that you are using your entire lungs when you breathe. You can also try placing a hand on your stomach and breathing so that your stomach expands. This will help to ensure that you are taking full breaths.

Pursed-lip breathing
Pursed-lip breathing is a type of deep breathing that can help to prevent mucus buildup and ease shortness of breath.

To do pursed-lip breathing:
1. Sit up straight with your shoulders relaxed. Place one hand on your stomach and the other on your chest.
2. Slowly breathe in through your nose for two counts, letting your stomach rise.
3. Purse your lips as if you are going to whistle and breathe out slowly for four counts.
4. Repeat this until you have breathed out all the air in your lungs.

Pursed-lip breathing can help to prevent mucus buildup by keeping the airways open and allowing the lungs to empty fully.

Additionally, it can help to ease shortness of breath by increasing oxygen levels in the blood. Pursed-lip breathing is a simple and effective way to improve lung function and respiratory health.

Incentive spirometry
Incentive spirometry is a deep breathing exercise that uses a

machine to help you breathe correctly. This can help to improve lung function and prevent exacerbations. The machine has a mouthpiece that you breathe into, and a ball that rises as you inhale. There are also markings on the ball, so you can see how much air you are taking in.

In order to get the full benefit of incentive spirometry, it is important to use the correct technique. You should take a deep breath in, hold it for a few seconds, and then breathe out slowly. It is also important to do the exercises regularly, as this will help to improve your lung function in the long term.

Yoga
Yoga is an ancient practice that combines physical and mental exercises to promote well-being. While it is often thought of as a way to improve flexibility, yoga can also be beneficial for lung health.

Studies have shown that yoga can help to improve lung function and ease shortness of breath. In particular, deep breathing exercises can help to expand the lungs and increase their capacity.

Additionally, the relaxation techniques taught in yoga can help to reduce stress and tension, which can lead to improved breathing. While anyone can benefit from yoga, it is especially helpful for those who suffer from respiratory conditions such as asthma or COPD.

By incorporating yoga into your daily routine, you can help to improve your lung function and ease your shortness of breath.

Quit smoking
It is well-known that smoking is detrimental to one's health, but many people continue to smoke anyway. If you are one of those people, it is important to be aware of the risks. Smoking is the leading cause of bronchiectasis.

If you smoke, quitting is the best thing you can do for your health.

Quitting will improve your lung function and overall health. It may be difficult, but it is worth it. So if you smoke, make the decision to quit today. Your lungs will thank you for it.

Tai chi
Tai chi is a type of exercise that originated in China. It is based on the principle of yin and yang and involves slow, deliberate movements. Tai chi can be performed by people of all ages and levels of fitness and has a number of benefits.

For example, it can help to improve balance and coordination, and can also help to ease shortness of breath. Tai chi is a low-impact form of exercise, which means that it is gentle on the joints. It is also suitable for people who are not used to exercising regularly. If you are thinking of starting tai chi, please speak to your doctor first.

Pilates
Pilates is a type of exercise that helps improve core strength and flexibility. It can also ease shortness of breath. Pilates exercises are done by lying on a mat, using body weight for resistance. The exercises help develop strong abdominal muscles and a strong lower back. They also help improve posture and flexibility.

Many people who do Pilates say that they feel taller and have less pain in their back, hips, and knees. Pilates can be done at home with DVDs or online videos, or at a studio with an instructor. You can also find Pilates classes at some gyms or community centers.

Regular exercise can help to improve lung function and prevent exacerbations. It is important to talk to your doctor before starting any new exercise routine.

Step Three: Making Dietary Changes
A healthy diet is an important part of this treatment, as it can help to improve overall health and reduce inflammation. Including plenty of fruits, vegetables, and whole grains in the diet, and avoiding processed foods and sugary drinks, can help to make a

difference for people with bronchiectasis.

Eating more fruits and vegetables
Fruits and vegetables are packed with nutrients, vitamins, and minerals that can help keep your immune system strong. Vitamin C, for example, is a well-known antioxidant found in most fruits. Vitamin C helps to protect cells from damage. It can also help to fight off infection by stimulating the production of white blood cells. Other vitamins and minerals, such as zinc and vitamin E, also play an important role in maintaining a healthy immune system.

In addition, phytochemicals found in fruits and vegetables can also help to fight disease. For example, lycopene, a substance found in tomatoes, has been shown to reduce the risk of some types of cancer. So remember to include plenty of fruits and vegetables in your diet to help boost your immune system and fight off infection.

Eating foods rich in antioxidants
Foods rich in antioxidants, such as blueberries, kale, and spinach, are particularly beneficial, as they help to protect the lungs from damage.

Having bronchiectasis means that your airways are permanently damaged and widened. This makes it difficult for you to clear mucus from your lungs, which can lead to infection. Eating a healthy diet is important for people with bronchiectasis, as it can help to improve lung function and reduce inflammation.

By making sure that you eat a healthy diet, you will be helping to protect your lungs and improve your overall health.

Avoiding processed foods
Bronchiectasis can be a difficult condition to live with. There are a few things that you can do to make your symptoms more

manageable, though. One of those things is avoiding processed foods.

Processed foods are often high in sugar and additives that can worsen bronchiectasis symptoms. They can also be difficult to digest, which can put added stress on your lungs. Instead, focus on eating fresh, whole foods that are easy on your lungs and won't trigger a flare-up. This way, you'll be able to better control your symptoms and manage your bronchiectasis.

Avoiding dairy products
Bronchiectasis is a condition in which the airways become damaged, leading to difficulty breathing. The symptoms of bronchiectasis can be exacerbated by mucus buildup, and dairy products are a common culprit.

Milk and other dairy products contain a protein called casein, which can contribute to mucus production. In addition, dairy products are often high in saturated fats, which can also lead to mucus buildup.

For those with bronchiectasis, eliminating dairy products from their diet can help to reduce mucus production and make breathing easier.

Increasing your intake of omega-3 fatty acids
Bronchiectasis is often caused by inflammation, so increasing your intake of omega-3 fatty acids may help to improve your symptoms. Omega-3 fatty acids are found in fish, nuts, and seeds. These healthy fats help to reduce inflammation throughout the body, including in the lungs.

In addition, omega-3 fatty acids have been shown to improve lung function and bronchial clearance in people with bronchiectasis. So if you're looking to improve your Bronchiectasis symptoms, increasing your intake of omega-3 fatty acids is a good place to start.

Creating a meal plan every week

To help you keep track of your dietary changes, making meal plans will greatly benefit you. Below is a sample 7-day meal plan that you can either follow or modify, depending on your preference. Take note that you don't have to strictly prepare one recipe per meal. You can save leftovers and eat them for later.

Meal	Breakfast	Lunch	Dinner
Day 1	Blueberry Pancakes	Italian Sweet Pepper-Tomato Pasta	Crunchy Kale Chips
Day 2	Avocado Egg Toast	Crispy Pork Chop with Flavorful Brussels Sprouts	Clam Chowder and Croutons
Day 3	Toasted Muesli	One-Pot Beans and Zucchini Penne	Crunchy Popcorn Chicken
Day 4	Egg Roll Bowl	Vegetable Pasta in Avocado Sauce	Cinnamon and Orange Beef Stew
Day 5	Blackberry Cobbler	Tomato and Turkey Panini	Crunchy Popcorn Chicken
Day 6	Blueberry Pancakes	Seaweed Salad	Crispy Pork Chop with Flavorful Brussels Sprouts
Day 7	Toasted Muesli	One-Pot Beans and Zucchini Penne	Cinnamon and Orange Beef Stew

SAMPLE MEALS

Blueberry Pancakes

Ingredients:
- 3 omega-3 fresh eggs
- 1 tsp. cinnamon
- 1/2 cup of arrowroot powder
- 1/4 cup of coconut oil
- 1/4 cup walnuts, roughly chopped
- 1 pinch sea salt
- 1/2 tsp. of baking soda
- 1/2 tsp. of yeast
- 1/2 cup of coconut flour
- 1 tsp. vanilla extract
- 1/2 tbsp. lemon juice
- 1 pint blueberries

Instructions:
1. Whisk 3 eggs. Pour vanilla, lemon juice, and almond milk. Mix well.
2. In another bowl, combine arrowroot, salt, yeast, baking powder, cinnamon, and coconut flour. Add wet mixture to this mixture while whisking continuously.
3. Fold in the chopped walnuts.
4. Grease a saucepan over medium heat with coconut oil.
5. Once the oil is hot, scoop the mixture with a ladle, and pour the pancakes onto the saucepan. Cook until bubbles form. Repeat this step until the batter is consumed.
6. For the sauce, simmer blueberries in another saucepan.
7. Add 4 tsp. of water. Simmer for 10 minutes.
8. Pour the sauce over a stack of pancakes and serve.

<u>Avocado Egg Toast</u>

Instructions:
- 1/4 avocado
- 1/8 tsp. garlic powder
- 1/4 tsp. ground pepper
- 1 pc. fried egg
- 1 slice toasted whole-wheat bread
- Optional: 1 tbsp. scallion
- Optional: 1 tsp. sriracha

Instructions:

1. Mash the avocado together with the garlic powder and pepper in a bowl.

2. Put the mashed avocado on the toast.

3. Add the egg on top then garnish with scallion and sriracha.

4. Serve immediately.

Toasted Muesli

Ingredients:
- 4 cups oats
- 1-1/2 cups raw walnut
- 1/2 cup pepitas
- 1/2 cup raw sunflower seeds
- 1/4 cup honey
- 2 tbsp. olive oil
- 1-1/2 tsp. ground cardamom
- 1/2 tsp. salt
- 1 cup freeze-dried strawberries
- 1 cup freeze-dried blueberries
- non-dairy milk or yogurt

Instructions:
1. Preheat the oven. Bring it to 350°F.
2. Mix all the ingredients in a bowl except the non-dairy milk.
3. Put the mixture in a baking pan. Spread evenly.
4. Put it in the preheated oven then toast for 20 to 30 minutes. Do not let the seeds and nuts scorch.
5. Bring it out from the oven. Let it cool. then serve with non-dairy milk or yogurt.

Egg Roll Bowl

Ingredients:
- 1 package of defrosted egg roll wrappers, cut into 0.5x3-inch per piece
- 1.5 lbs. ground pork
- 3 small cloves of garlic, minced
- 2 tsp. fresh ginger, peeled and minced
- 1/2 cup vegetable or chicken broth
- 1/3 cup coconut aminos
- 1.5 tsp. toasted sesame oil
- 1 9-oz. package pre-shredded cabbage
- 3-4 green onions, chopped
- Sriracha sauce

Instructions:
1. Preheat the oven to 400°F.
2. Place wrappers on a baking sheet. Brush with a little olive oil.
3. Bake for about 5 minutes, or until golden brown.
4. In a large pan, heat 1 tbsp. of oil over medium-high heat.
5. Add raw meat. Cook for about 4-5 minutes, or until golden brown.
6. Drain or pat with a paper towel after removing from the pan.
7. Raw meat is browned in a pan
8. In the same pan, turn heat to medium. Add garlic and ginger, stir occasionally for about a minute.
9. Add cabbage slaw mix and most of the green onions. Cook for around 3 minutes until softened.
10. Add broth, coconut amino, and sesame oil. Stir well.
11. Put everything in a bowl. Top it with toasted egg roll wrappers, Sriracha, and leftover green onions.

Blackberry Cobbler

Ingredients:
- 2 tbsp. organic coconut oil, with an additional amount for greasing
- 1/4 cup arrowroot flour
- 12 oz. blackberries
- 1/4 cup raw honey
- 3 tbsp. water
- 1/4 tsp. salt
- 1-1/4 tsp. lemon juice
- 3/4 tsp. baking soda
- 1/4 cup coconut flour

Instructions:
1. Preheat the oven to 300°F.
2. Use coconut oil to grease an 8×8 baking dish.
3. Place blackberries at the bottom of the pan, ensuring that they are placed evenly.
4. Place remaining ingredients in a food processor. Pulse at medium speed until thoroughly combined and then spread over blackberries.
5. Bake for 35 to 40 minutes or until the top turns golden brown.
6. Serve and enjoy.

Italian Sweet Pepper-Tomato Pasta

Ingredients:
- 2 small red onions, diced
- 3 tbsp. olive oil
- 3/4 tsp. garlic powder
- 1 vegetable stock cube
- 1/2 tsp. sea salt
- 1 tsp. cumin
- 1/4 tsp. cinnamon
- 1 tbsp. dried basil
- 1 cup of fresh parsley
- 1 tbsp. dried oregano
- 2 sprigs fresh oregano
- 1/2 black pepper
- 1 cup canned Roma tomatoes
- 1 tbsp. dried cilantro
- 2 red tomatoes, chopped
- 1 cup baby sweet peppers
- 1/2 lb. pasta

Instructions:
1. In a large pan, heat the olive oil for 30 seconds. Add onions, spices, and vegetable stock.
2. Add in the tomatoes, herbs, and pepper; simmer for about 15 minutes.
3. Once tomatoes are soft, mash with a fork or transfer to a food processor.
4. In the same pan, add water and pasta; cook until al dente.
5. Serve on a plate, top with extra basil leaf garnishing.

Vegetable Pasta in Avocado Sauce

Ingredients:
Zucchini Pasta
- 2 zucchini
- 3 cups red and yellow cherry tomatoes
- 4 oz. pasta

Avocado Sauce
- 1/2 cup fresh parsley
- 1 tbsp. miso paste
- 1 garlic clove
- 1 avocado
- 1/4 cup olive oil
- 4 green onions
- 1/2 tsp. salt
- juice from 1 lemon
- ground pepper, to taste

Instructions:
1. To make the avocado sauce, use a blender to pulse all ingredients until smooth. Set aside.
2. In a large skillet over high heat, drizzle olive oil and cook cherry tomatoes until skin loosens. Season with ground pepper and salt.
3. In the same skillet, add the zucchini, and avocado sauce; toss to combine.
4. To serve, season with ground pepper and salt to taste; garnish with extra tomatoes.

One-Pot Beans and Zucchini Penne

Ingredients:
- 8 oz. dry penne
- 1/4 cup onion, diced
- 1/4 cup water
- 3 cloves garlic, pressed
- 1 tbsp. dried oregano
- 1 tbsp. dried basil
- 3 zucchinis, cubed
- 2 cans Great Northern beans, rinsed and drained
- 2 28-oz. cans tomatoes, diced
- sea salt
- ground pepper

Instructions:
1. Pour 1/4 cup water in a large pot.
2. Add garlic and onions.
3. Water-fry for 3 to 5 minutes.
4. Add all other ingredients and cook until pasta is al dente, stirring frequently.
5. Adjust seasoning to taste. Serve while warm.

Clam Chowder and Croutons

Ingredients:
- 1 lb. potatoes
- 1 medium onion, diced finely
- 2 tbsp. unsalted butter
- 2 cups chicken broth
- 2 celery stalks
- 2 cans clams in juice
- 1 cup heavy cream
- 3 tbsp. all-purpose flour
- 2 bay leaves
- 2 celery stalks
- 1 cup heavy cream
- salt
- pepper

For the croutons:
- 3 tbsp. parsley
- 1/2 baguette
- pepper
- salt

Instructions:
1. In a large pot, add the onions, butter, and celery. Sauté until soft.
2. In the same pot, add the flour, stock, clams juice, heavy cream, potatoes, and bay leaves.
3. Simmer all the ingredients until thick. Reduce heat and cook for about 20 minutes.
4. Once the potatoes are tender, add the clams. Season with pepper and salt.
5. Meanwhile, in a large skillet, toss the cubed baguettes with the butter.
6. Toast and brown the bread for 3 minutes. Add parsley then season with salt and pepper.
7. Serve while hot.

Tomato and Turkey Panini

Ingredients:
- 3 tbsp. fat-reduced mayonnaise
- 1 tsp. lemon juice
- 2 tbsp. plain, non-fat yogurt
- freshly ground pepper
- 2 tbsp. shredded parmesan cheese
- 8 pcs. sodium-reduced turkey, sliced thinly
- 2 tbsp. fresh basil, chopped finely
- 8 slices of tomato
- 2 tsp. canola oil

Instructions:
1. Combine parmesan, mayonnaise, yogurt, lemon juice, basil, and pepper in a bowl.
2. Spread 2 teaspoons of the mixture on each bread.
3. Divide tomato and turkey slices evenly among the four slices of bread. Top each with the remaining bread.
4. Heat a teaspoon of oil in a skillet over medium heat.
5. Place two panini in the pan. Place the skillet on top of the panini. Use the cans to weigh it down.
6. Cook the panini until they turn golden on one side, which may take about a couple of minutes.
7. Reduce the heat to low and flow the panini.
8. Repeat the same process on the other side. Cook the remaining Panini.
9. Serve and enjoy immediately.

Crunchy Popcorn Chicken

Ingredients:
- 1 lb. skinless chicken cubes
- 1/2 cup cornstarch
- 1/2 tsp. onion powder
- 1/2 tsp. garlic powder
- 1 cup unsweetened coconut milk
- 1/2 tsp. paprika
- 3 cups crushed corn flakes
- 1/4 tsp. cayenne pepper
- 1/4 tsp. black pepper
- 1 tsp. pickle juice

Instructions:
1. Pour the cornstarch on a plate and set aside.
2. In a bowl, mix the coconut milk and pickle juice.
3. Take a plastic bag and add corn flakes along with the spices. Crush the flakes and pour them onto a plate.
4. Coat the chicken cubes with cornstarch and then dip them into coconut milk. Now, roll them over the flake crumbs. Repeat the process with all the chicken cubes.
5. Take out the air fryer basket and lightly coat with cooking spray. Place the chicken cubes in a single layer.
6. Bake the cubes at 400°F for 10 minutes.
7. Once they turn golden, take them out.
8. Serve hot.

Crispy Pork Chop with Flavorful Brussels Sprouts

Ingredients:
- 8 oz. pork chop, bone-in and center-cut
- 6 oz. Brussels sprouts
- 1/2 tsp. ground black pepper
- 1 tsp. olive oil
- 1 tsp. maple syrup
- 1 tsp. Dijon mustard
- cooking spray

Instructions:
1. In a bowl, put the pork chop and coat it lightly with cooking spray. Add half of the black pepper over it.
2. Take another bowl and add the oil along with maple syrup, dijon mustard, and remaining black pepper. Whisk them well.
3. In the mixture, add Brussels sprouts and toss them.
4. Place the marinated pork chop on one side of the air fryer basket. On the other side, place the coated sprouts.
5. Heat the air fryer to 400°F.
6. Place the basket and cook it until the pork turns golden brown.
7. After it turns golden, cook it for another 10 minutes to make it more tender.

Cinnamon and Orange Beef Stew

Ingredients:
- 2 lbs. beef
- 3 cups beef broth
- 2 whole bay leaves
- 1 tsp. sage
- 1 tsp. rosemary
- 1 tsp. soy sauce
- 1 tsp. fish sauce
- 3 tbsp. coconut oil
- Orange zest
- 1 onion, chopped
- Orange juice
- 1 tsp. salt
- 1-1/2 tsp. black pepper
- 2 tsp. erythritol
- 2 tsp. ground cinnamon
- 2 tbsp. Apple cider vinegar
- 1 tbsp. fresh thyme
- 2-1/2 tsp. minced garlic

Instructions:
1. Cut vegetables into dice and the meat into cubes.
2. Heat the oil in a skillet and add meat. Do this in sets. Cook until brown.
3. After the last batch, add vegetables and cook for 2-3 minutes.
4. Deglaze the pan by adding orange juice.
5. Add all the remaining ingredients, except for the thyme, sage, and rosemary.
6. Cook for 1-2 minutes and transfer the mixture to a crockpot.
7. Cook on high for 2-3 hours.
8. Gently open the crockpot and add rosemary, sage, and thyme.
9. Cook for another 2 hours on high.
10. Serve while hot.

Seaweed Salad

Ingredients:
- 4 tsp. fish sauce
- 2 oz. dried seaweed such as wakame, arame, dulse, or agar
- 2 green onions, finely chopped
- 1 tsp. fresh ginger juice
- 2 tbsp. coconut water vinegar
- 2 tsp. honey
- 2 cups cucumber, finely sliced
- 1/4 cup fresh lemon juice
- 2 cups daikon radish or Japanese turnip, finely sliced

Instructions:
1. Mix together the honey, coconut water vinegar, lemon juice, fish sauce, and ginger juice to create a salad dressing.
2. Immerse the seaweed in cold water for at least 5 minutes, or until it is adequately soft.
3. Rinse and drain after. Chop if the pieces are too big.
4. Combine the rehydrated seaweed with turnips, radish, cucumber, and dressing.
5. Top with green onions as a garnish.
6. Serve and enjoy.

Crunchy Kale Chips

Ingredients:
- 1 large bunch lacinato kale, destemmed and cut into uniform pieces
- 1 cup cashews, soaked and drained
- 3 cloves garlic
- 1 tbsp. tamari sauce
- 1/4 cup nutritional yeast
- 2 tbsp. water

Instructions:
1. Blend cashews with a blender, creating a thick paste.
2. Not including the kale and water, add all the ingredients into the blender and blend them well.
3. Gradually add water to make the mixture thick and creamy.
4. Pour the mixture over the kale. Coat the paste on the leaves with your hands.
5. Place the coated kale leaves in a single layer on the air fryer's basket. Bake the leaves for 10-15 minutes at 350°F, or until the chips turn crispy.
6. Serve and enjoy immediately.

CONCLUSION

In summary, bronchiectasis is a chronic lung condition that can be improved by managing symptoms through natural methods and diet. People with bronchiectasis often experience shortness of breath, coughing up mucus, and fatigue. These symptoms can be managed by avoiding triggers, such as cigarette smoke and air pollution, and by staying hydrated.

Additionally, a nutritious diet rich in antioxidants and anti-inflammatory foods can help to reduce symptoms and improve lung function. With proper management, people with bronchiectasis can enjoy a good quality of life.

If you or someone you know has bronchiectasis, it is important to seek medical attention and follow the treatment plan prescribed by a healthcare professional. Additionally, self-care measures, such as those outlined in this article, can help to reduce symptoms and improve overall health.

FAQ ABOUT BRONCHIECTASIS

What is bronchiectasis?
Bronchiectasis is a chronic lung condition in which the airways become damaged and widened. This damage leads to difficulty clearing mucus from the lungs, which can lead to infection. Bronchiectasis can be caused by a variety of conditions, including allergies, autoimmune disorders, and infections.

What are the symptoms of bronchiectasis?
The most common symptoms of bronchiectasis include shortness of breath, coughing up mucus, and fatigue. People with bronchiectasis may also experience wheezing, chest pain, and difficulty sleeping.

How is bronchiectasis diagnosed?
Bronchiectasis is usually diagnosed by a lung specialist (pulmonologist) after reviewing your medical history and conducting a physical exam. A chest X-ray or CT scan may also be ordered to confirm the diagnosis.

How is bronchiectasis treated?
There is no cure for bronchiectasis, but treatment can help to improve symptoms and prevent complications. Treatment typically involves a combination of medications, such as antibiotics and inhalers, and self-care measures, such as quitting

smoking and staying hydrated. In some cases, surgery may also be necessary to remove damaged tissue.

What is the long-term outlook for people with bronchiectasis?
Most people with bronchiectasis can expect to live a normal life span with proper treatment. However, complications from bronchiectasis, such as lung infections, can be serious and even life-threatening. With proper treatment and self-care, most people with bronchiectasis can enjoy a good quality of life.

What are some self-care measures I can take to manage my bronchiectasis?
There are a number of self-care measures you can take to manage your bronchiectasis and reduce your symptoms. These include:
- avoiding triggers, such as cigarette smoke and air pollution
- staying hydrated
- eating a nutritious diet
- exercising regularly
- getting vaccinated against influenza and pneumonia
- practicing good hygiene, such as washing your hands often and avoiding close contact with people who are sick.

How can I prevent bronchiectasis?
Unfortunately, there is no sure way to prevent bronchiectasis. However, there are a few things you can do to reduce your risk:
- quit smoking
- avoid exposure to lung irritants, such as air pollution and chemical fumes
- treat any underlying conditions, such as allergies or infections
- get vaccinated against influenza and pneumonia.

What are the complications of bronchiectasis?
Complications from bronchiectasis can be serious and even life-threatening. The most common complications include lung infections, such as pneumonia, and difficulty breathing. Other complications include heart failure, lung cancer, and death.

When should I see a doctor?
If you think you may have bronchiectasis, it is important to see a doctor as soon as possible. Bronchiectasis is a chronic condition that can worsen over time, so early diagnosis and treatment are essential.

KEY TAKEAWAYS

- Bronchiectasis is a chronic lung condition in which the airways become damaged and widened.

- The most common symptoms of bronchiectasis include shortness of breath, coughing up mucus, and fatigue.

- There is no cure for bronchiectasis, but treatment can help to improve symptoms and prevent complications.

- Most people with bronchiectasis can expect to live a normal life span with proper treatment.

- Self-care measures, such as staying hydrated and avoiding triggers, can help to manage bronchiectasis.

- Bronchiectasis can lead to serious complications, such as lung infections and heart failure. If you think you may have bronchiectasis, it is important to see a doctor as soon as possible.

REFERENCES

"Bronchiectasis." NHS.UK, 19 Oct. 2017, https://www.nhs.uk/conditions/bronchiectasis/. Accessed 28 July 2022.

"Bronchiectasis; Causes, Symptoms, Treatment & Prevention." Cleveland Clinic, https://my.clevelandclinic.org/health/diseases/21144-bronchiectasis. Accessed 28 July 2022.

Bronchiectasis - What Is Bronchiectasis? | NHLBI, NIH. https://www.nhlbi.nih.gov/health/bronchiectasis. Accessed 29 July 2022.

Donovan, John. "Bronchiectasis." WebMD, https://www.webmd.com/lung/what-is-bronchiectasis. Accessed 28 July 2022.

Yadav, Asha, et al. "Effect of Yoga Regimen on Lung Functions Including Diffusion Capacity in Coronary Artery Disease Patients: A Randomized Controlled Study." International Journal of Yoga, vol. 8, no. 1, 2015, pp. 62–67. PubMed Central, https://doi.org/10.4103/0973-6131.146067. Accessed 28 July 2022.

Made in United States
Troutdale, OR
12/17/2023